Angina
Second Edition

W0018841

Angina

SECOND EDITION

Graham Jackson FRCP, FESC
Consultant Cardiologist
Guy's Hospital
London, UK

MARTIN DUNITZ

Although every effort has been made to ensure that the drug doses and other information are presented accurately in this publication, the ultimate responsibility rests with the prescribing physician. Neither the publishers nor the author can be held responsible for errors or for any consequences arising from the use of information contained herein.

© Martin Dunitz Ltd 1991, 1995

First published in the United Kingdom
in 1991 by
Martin Dunitz Ltd
7– 9 Pratt Street
London NW1 0AE

First edition 1991
Second edition 1995

Reprinted 1995

ISBN 1-85317-208-1

Printed and bound in Spain by Cayfosa

Contents

Dedication
For Maggie, Keira and Matthew

Introduction

Angina pectoris is a common symptom, usually reflecting coronary artery disease (CAD). As the location and extent of the coronary disease, along with the quality of left ventricular (LV) function, determine prognosis it is important to make an accurate diagnosis as soon as possible. Management is not designed only to relieve symptoms, and thereby improve the quality of life; but by appropriately timed non-invasive and invasive investigations we need to identify those at most risk so that we can select optimal therapy which will also lengthen life.

This handbook is meant to be practical and help answer the following questions:

- Is it angina?

- How should I treat it?

- Who should be referred?

- What tests are needed and when?

- What is the place of drugs, angioplasty and surgery?

This second edition has been reviewed and expanded with regard to the increasing importance of managing hyperlipidaemia, diagnosing and treating CAD in women and managing chest pain with normal coronary arteries. In addition the roles of angioplasty, stent insertion and coronary bypass surgery have been updated and compared.

Background

Incidence
Definitions
Diagnosis of chest pain
Stable angina: clinical evaluation
Investigations

Incidence

Coronary artery disease is responsible for over 450 deaths per day in the UK. Each year in the UK alone 320 000 people consult for angina and 300 000 experience myocardial infarcts.

Coronary artery disease is an equal opportunity killer affecting postmenopausal and premenopausal women as well as men. In the USA in 1989 cardiovascular disease claimed over 940 000 lives and ischaemic heart disease accounted for 500 000 deaths, of which 240 000 occurred in women. In contrast breast cancer claims 43 000 of women's lives and lung cancer 51 000 lives whilst stroke claims 88 000 lives.

One in three men and women over 65 years of age has some form of cardiovascular disease. Below 65, women have approximately half the rate of men:

> age 40–44 years 1 in 8 men, 1 in 16 women;
> age 45–50 years 1 in 6 men, 1 in 12 women;
> age 45–64 years 1 in 5 men, 1 in 9 women.

Though overall death rates from cardiovascular disease are slowly declining, the number of women dying from cardiovascular disease is increasing.

Cardiovascular disease is therefore a major concern for men and women and the leading cause of death for both. It is not a matter of whether women can develop CAD — but when.

It is important that both doctors and women become aware of the possibility of CAD developing and treat the potential for ischaemia as vigorously in women as in men.

Cost

The indirect costs of CAD are significant, with 12% of working days lost in the UK through sickness being due to CAD — about £1.8 billion annually in lost earnings. The annual direct cost to the NHS in 1989 was estimated at £500 million. In the USA the annual cost is approximately $117 billion.

Age

As the population ages, the incidence of angina as a manifestation of CAD will increase. In addition, by educating the public and increasing awareness of CAD there should be an increasing workload and the need for precise investigation and diagnosis will become even more important.

- Coronary artery disease is the leading cause of death in men *and* women.
- Angina is common.
- Angina will become more common as the population is aging.
- Effective strategies for diagnosis, investigation and treatment are essential.

Definitions

Stable angina

Stable angina is ischaemic cardiac pain, which may be perceived in many ways (Table 1), that is brought on by effort and relieved by rest. It will have been present for several weeks or longer, precipitated by predictable factors and relieved promptly by rest and/or sublingual nitrates. It will not have worsened recently in terms of severity of attacks, increasing frequency of attacks or attacks at rest (see Table 2).

Angina is a clinical diagnosis based on the doctor's interpretation of the patient's story. A good history needs no confirmatory tests but tests will be needed to evaluate risk and optimize management.

Cardiac	Non-cardiac
Tightness	Sharp (not severe)
Pressure	Knife-like
Weight	Stabbing
Constriction	'Like a stitch'
Ache	'Like a needle'
Dull	Pricking feeling
Squeezing feeling	Shooting
Soreness	Reproduced by pressure or position
Crushing	Can walk around with it
'Like a band'	Continuous: 'It's there all day'
Breathless (tightness)	

Table 1
Chest pain characteristics.

1 'Ordinary physical activity does not cause angina': this includes walking and climbing stairs. Angina with strenuous or rapid or prolonged exertion at work or recreation.

2 'Slight limitation of ordinary activity': this includes walking or climbing stairs rapidly, walking uphill, walking or stair-climbing after meals, or in cold, or in wind, or under emotional stress, or only during the few hours after awakening; walking more than two blocks on the level and climbing more than one flight of ordinary stairs at a normal pace and in normal conditions.

3 'Marked limitation of ordinary physical activity': this includes walking one to two blocks on the level and climbing one flight of stairs in normal conditions and at normal pace.

4 'Inability to carry on any physical activity without discomfort — anginal syndrome may be present at rest'.

Table 2
Grading of angina of effort by the Canadian Cardiovascular Society.

Unstable angina

The term 'unstable angina' describes a clinical presentation between stable angina and myocardial infarction; it may move in either direction. Clinically the presentation can be divided into three groups:

- Effort angina of recent onset (less than 1 month) — no previous angina

- Changing pattern of angina with stable angina increasing in frequency and/or severity

- Angina at rest for no obvious reason.

Other names for unstable angina include the intermediate coronary syndrome, pre-infarction angina, crescendo angina, acute coronary insufficiency and accelerated angina.

Diagnosis of chest pain

There are many causes of chest pain. Clinically we are concerned with differentiating angina from chest wall pain, oesophageal pain or functional pain perhaps linked to hyperventilation.

Nature of the pain

Ischaemic pain can be defined by asking the following questions:

- Site — Where is the pain?
- Radiation — Where does it go?
- Character — What does it feel like?
- Causes — What brings it on?
- Relief — What do you do when you have the pain?

Site
The site of pain may be retrosternal: this can be localized but is more usually spread across the chest.

The patient may place his hand across the chest (Figure 1) or clench his fist (Figure 2), emphasizing the squeezing constriction sometimes felt.

The pain is only very rarely localized (Figure 3) — this is usually muscular chest wall pain.

Radiation
Pain usually radiates out from the chest rather than into the chest. Presentation in referral sites only is unusual but can be dangerous, particularly if there is severe epigastric pain, which may lead to a gastroscopy or laparotomy (Table 3).

Figure 1
The patient may draw the flat of his hand across the chest.

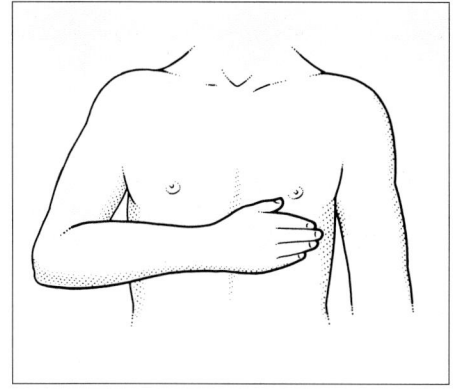

Figure 2
Clenched fist in the centre (Levine's sign) illustrating the constriction or tightness felt.

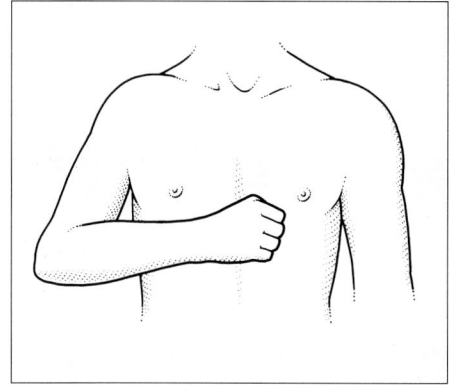

Figure 3
The patient almost never points to the pain as if localized.

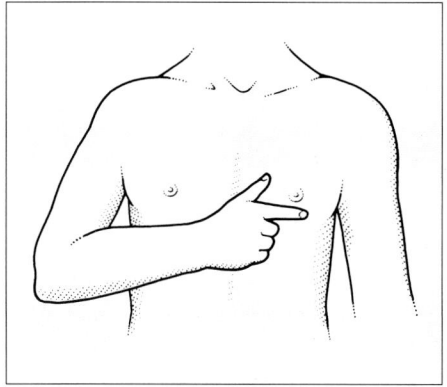

Location of pain	Sole involvement (per cent)	Partial involvement (per cent)
Anterior chest	34.0	96.0
Left arm (upper)	0.7	30.7
Left arm (lower)	1.3	29.3
Right arm (upper)	0	10.0
Right arm (lower)	0	13.3
Back	0.7	16.7
Epigastrium	0.7	3.3
Forehead	0	6.0
Neck	2.0	22.0
Chin and perioral area	0	8.7

Table 3
Sites of anginal pain in 150 successive ambulatory patients.

The commonest sites are shown in Figure 4:

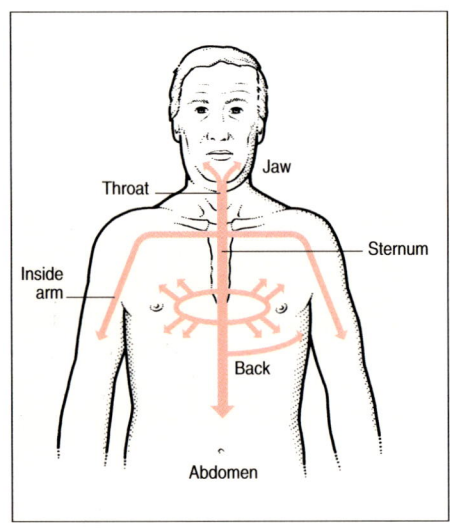

Figure 4
Site and radiation of cardiac pain.

- Neck and throat: patients present with a 'choking', 'strangling', or 'suffocating' feeling
- Jaw: 'toothache', 'dentures a problem'
- Left arm, right arm or both: pain is usually felt down the *inside* under the axilla to the inner two fingers
- Abdomen: 'indigestion'
- Back: 'arthritis'
- Site of previous injury (eg, fractured arm, severe spondylosis, carious tooth).

Anyone presenting with epigastric pain who is over 40 years of age and at cardiac risk (eg, smoker, hypertensive, male, diabetic) should have an ECG and an index of suspicion for a cardiac cause, even if the story strongly suggests a gastric problem.

Character

The sensation may be so mild that it is often dismissed by the patient as an ache rather than a pain. The commonest features are summarized in Table 1. Of note:

- Tightness is often perceived as breathlessness
- The pain usually builds up rather than being maximal at its onset
- Sharp, knife-like pain of sudden onset is not cardiac
- Beware local dialects — for example 'sharp' can sometimes mean 'severe' not 'knife-like'
- Watch the patient's hands as he talks — they often tell the story for him (Figures 1–3)
- If the patient is breathless ask what this means — is it a tightness or a winded feeling?

Causes

Angina is brought on by an increase in oxygen demand that cannot be met by supply.

With a supply and demand problem caused by obstructive CAD any factor increasing heart rate (ie, demand) at the expense of supply (shorter diastole — the coronaries fill in diastole) can induce pain.

The commonest causes are:

- Exertion: inclines, and stairs in particular
- Emotion: especially anger and anxiety
- A large meal: cardiac output rises 20 per cent
- Temperature change
- Windy weather
- Exciting films on TV: so-called 'match of the day' angina
- Vivid dreams: particularly if these are frightening
- Sexual intercourse: especially if this is extramarital or casual.

The above may be additive (eg, walking the dog in windy weather after a meal).

Post-prandial angina
This is angina within 30 minutes of a meal. It appears to be a marker of severity of disease and is more often associated with unstable angina. Particularly in patients with a previous myocardial infarct, it suggests severe coronary disease and should serve as an indication for early angiography.

Chest pain in women
Though chest pain in women is common, it is often atypical and difficult to pin down. With the lower prevalence of disease in younger women the history and also exercise ECGs are more likely to be false positive for CAD. Approximately 40 per cent of women with chest pain have normal coronary arteries (NCA) with the only factor predicting CAD being diabetes. In spite of NCA an appreciable number of women continue to experience

symptoms which often prove difficult to manage (see page 75). Where symptoms are atypical or minimal and/or where doubts exist, ie, where the doctor cannot say whether the patient is normal or not, further tests are required.

Relief
Slowing the heart rate by rest or relaxation will reduce demand. For example, the patient may walk slowly or sit down. Glyceryl trinitrate (GTN) relieves by vasodilatation, reducing demand. Relief is rapid — usually less than 10 minutes.

Pain relieved previously by GTN which now lengthens to 30 minutes may reflect unstable angina or infarction.

Unstable angina

Unstable angina may be new or worsening angina. Angina is noted at rest or minimal activity, and exercise tolerance may be suddenly and dramatically reduced.

It is still usually relieved by GTN; but needs hospital care.

Variant angina

Variant angina is also known as 'Prinzmetal's angina'. It is caused by spasm on a fixed coronary lesion or occasionally spasm when the coronary arteries are normal. It occurs:

- Usually at rest
- In response to cold
- Rarely on exercise
- At a consistent time of day — usually night or early morning
- Often with the sensation of palpitations.

The presence of ST elevation during ischaemia separates it from the more usual ST depression of other forms of angina.

Uncommon angina presentations

'Second wind angina' is the ability to walk off the pain, especially if the exercise is pleasurable (eg, golf).

'Tobacco angina' is the pain with cigarettes or, rarely, cigar smoking.

In angina decubitus the pain is worse when the patient lies down in bed. This is rare: perhaps dreams, or a cold bedroom or cold sheets are the cause (it is not due to syphilis, as was originally taught).

Pain of myocardial infarction

Pain from myocardial infarction lasts longer than angina — usually over 30 minutes, and is severe and retrosternal. It is characterized by pallor, perspiration, nausea and vomiting.

The pain is not relieved but may be modified by GTN.

Differential diagnosis

From the cardiac point of view there are two important differential diagnoses: acute pericarditis and dissecting aortic aneurysm. Non-cardiac causes of chest pain include pain secondary to pulmonary disease, gastrointestinal problems, musculoskeletal pain and functional chest pain (Table 4).

Oesophageal

Not usually exertional. Rarely radiates to left arm. Worse when lying flat or after a large meal. Relieved by belching, standing, antacids but also by GTN and calcium antagonists.

Pericarditis

Sharp pain worse on inspiration and lying flat. Relieved by shallow breathing and standing. Often pyrexial. Rub may be audible.

Pulmonary

Pleuritic pain, worse with breathing, often localized. Frequent cough or haemoptysis. Rub audible.

Musculoskeletal

Positional, localized, reproduced by pressure. Sharp, suddenly severe. May be tightness due to pectoral spasm. May be deep to the breast in women.

Functional

Hyperventilation. Patient easily breathless, frequent sighs, anxious, often young woman. Musculoskeletal pain may be associated.

Mitral valve prolapse

Mostly atypical but some typical pains and more common in younger women who may also hyperventilate. Frequently pain after exercise when fatigued.

Dissecting aortic aneurysm

Very severe pain to the back. At its most severe at its onset. May radiate to the lower abdomen, thighs and hips. Not affected by posture.

Table 4
Some differential features of chest pain.

Stable angina: clinical evaluation

Aetiology

Obstructive CAD is the commonest cause of angina pectoris. Other conditions with or without coexistent CAD should be considered:

- Coronary spasm: this usually occurs as rest pain
- Aortic stenosis: the patient is usually over 60 years of age
- Aortic incompetence: the patient is usually over 60 years of age
- LV hypertrophy: this occurs with hypertension and cardiomyopathy
- Anaemia
- Thyrotoxicosis
- Rapid or slow arrhythmias: these occur particularly in the elderly (atrial fibrillation)
- Severe mitral stenosis: a very rare cause
- Primary pulmonary hypertension: this is very rare also.

Examination

Usually no abnormality is found on clinical examination. Careful assessment may identify diagnostic clues:

- Nicotine-stained fingers or smell of tobacco
- Anaemia
- Premature arcus senilis in a patient less than 40 years old
- Xanthomas on the hands, elbows, knees or ankles indicate familial hypercholesterolaemia
- Xanthelasma is surprisingly non-specific.

The commonest auscultatory finding is a IVth heart sound (listen with bell at apex) reflecting reduced ventricular compliance. Also look for:

- Murmurs, which may be a sign of aortic and mitral valve disease
- Apical dyskinesia, indicating LV ischaemia or infarction
- Hypertension
- Isolated systolic hypertension: think also of aortic regurgitation
- Carotid or femoral bruits
- Peripheral pulses, which may be absent especially in diabetics or heavy smokers.
- Signs of diabetes.

A practical checklist is given in Table 5.

Table 5
Examination checklist.

Sign	Location	Comment
Xanthoma	Hands, elbows, knees	Hyperlipidaemia
Xanthelasma	Eyelids	Non-specific
Arcus senilis	Eyes	Non-specific over 40 years of age
IVth heart sound	Apex (turn to left side)	Reduced ventricular compliance
Immediate diastolic murmur	Third/fourth left intercostal space, patient leaning forward	Aortic incompetence
Ejection systolic murmur	Apex, second right intercostal space, neck	Aortic stenosis
Late or pansystolic murmur	Apex to axilla	Mitral regurgitation
Bruits	Both carotid and femoral arteries	Peripheral arterial disease

Patients with severe symptoms in spite of medical therapy have selected themselves for further investigations with a view to angioplasty (percutaneous transluminal coronary angioplasty, PTCA) or surgery (coronary artery bypass grafting, CABG). Unfortunately those with mild symptoms may have severe CAD and we need to identify them.

Three questions therefore need to be answered:

- Who is at risk?

- How do we identify him/her?

- Can we modify the risk?

Who is at risk?

Several studies have now been performed comparing surgery with medical treatment. These involved vein grafts rather than the now-preferred mammary artery conduits.

The Veterans Administration Study 1970–1974*

In the study group there was a high operative mortality of 5.8 per cent: this was in the early days of surgery, and there was therefore a lack of expertise. There was also vein patency of 69 per cent at one year, again reflecting technical limitations. In spite of this, surgery is better for left main stem disease.

There was limited medical therapy, as the new generation of drugs was not available.

* Murphy ML, Hultgren DN, Detre K et al, *Treatment of chronic stable angina: a preliminary report of survival data of the randomized Veterans Administration Co-operative Study*, N Engl J Med *(1977)* **297***: 621–7.*

The European Coronary Surgery Study 1973–1976*
The study group covered mild to moderate angina.

Better medical therapy with beta-blockade was available but not standardized. Operative mortality — at 3.6 per cent — was still high. Vein patency was 77 per cent at l8 months.

At 5 years 7.6 per cent of those undergoing surgery died, as opposed to 16.2 per cent of those undergoing medical treatment — a highly significant 53 per cent reduction. There was impressive benefit with left main stem disease (Figure 5) and 3-vessel disease (Figure 6); and there was also benefit for 2-vessel disease if one lesion was in the proximal left anterior descending (LAD) artery. There was more benefit if the resting and exercise ECG had been abnormal.

Figure 5
European Coronary Surgery Study: improved survival 5 years after CABG in patients with left main stem disease (LMD). S: surgery; M: medical treatment.

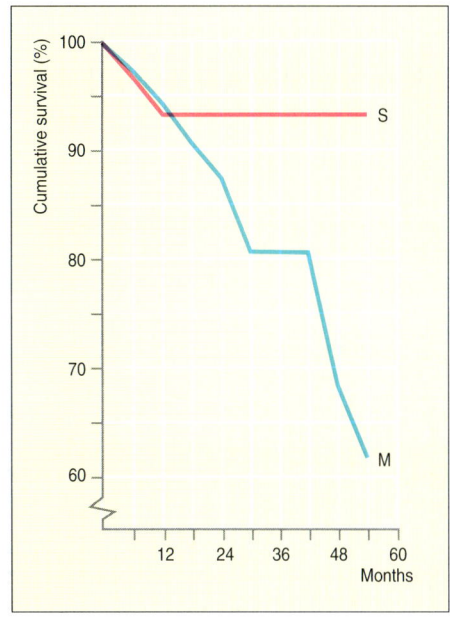

* European Coronary Surgery Study Group, Longterm results of a prospective randomised study of coronary artery bypass surgery in stable angina pectoris, Lancet (1982) **ii**: 1173–80.

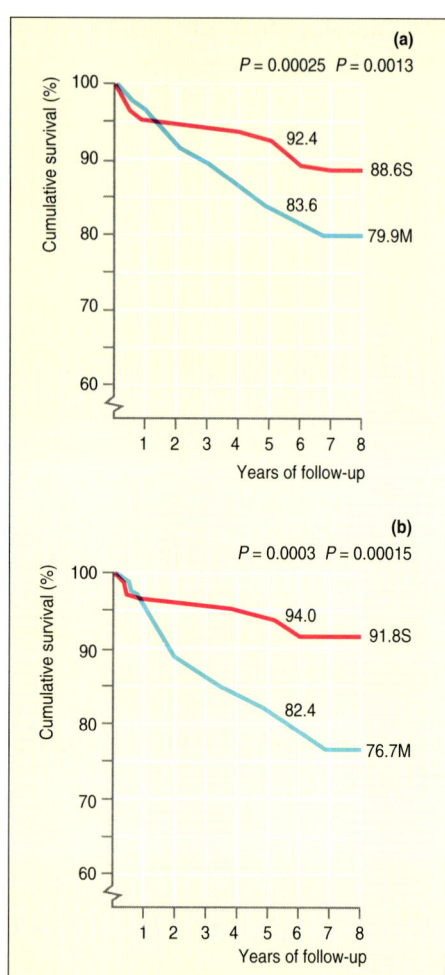

Figure 6
European Coronary Surgery Study Group: survival curves for randomized medical (M) and surgical (S) groups in the total population (a) and in the subset of patients (b) with 3-vessel disease.

The Coronary Artery Surgery Study (CASS)*

The study group was American. Left main stem disease was excluded. The study included no angina and very minimal

* CASS principal investigators and their associates, Coronary Artery Surgery Study (CASS): a randomised trial of coronary artery bypass surgery survival data, Circulation *(1983)* **68**: 939–50.

angina cases. Of 16 626 assessed only 780 were entered (Figure 7), which meant that the study was very selective!

Figure 7
Allocation of patients in Coronary Artery Surgery Study registry at randomizing sites: reasons for exclusion from study. Width is proportional to the number of patients in each category. LMCA: left main coronary artery; CHF: congestive heart failure.

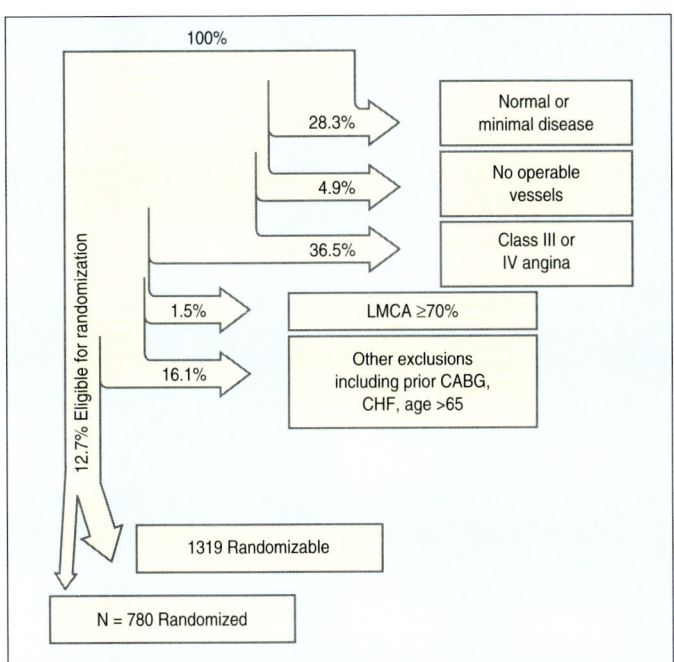

At 5 years 92 per cent of those undergoing medical and 95 per cent of those undergoing surgical treatment survived: this is not a significant divergence. Operative mortality was 1.4 per cent, which is the current figure. Graft patency at 60 days was 90 per cent.

One should note that in the medical group only 43 per cent used beta-blockers. Surgery was better at 6 years if there was 3-vessel disease and reduced LV function.

Rationalizing the trials; modifying the risk

It is important to note that different patients are being evaluated and so a combined message becomes possible based on who is at risk and who will benefit.

- An abnormal exercise test may identify someone at risk

- If there is left main stem disease there will be a surgical benefit

- If there is 3-vessel disease, with and without good LV function, there will be surgical benefit

- If there is 2-vessel disease including proximal LAD disease there will be surgical benefit

- If there are minimal symptoms and a normal or slightly abnormal exercise ECG, medical therapy is indicated.

One should note that in Europe only higher-risk patients are selected and operated on: I believe this is the correct strategy.

It is also important to note that the latter two trials were weighted against surgery: medical patients who needed surgery because of symptoms remained classed as 'medical'; and surgical patients who refused operation were still classed as 'surgical'.

Furthermore with the use of internal mammary artery conduits long-term graft patency rates have improved markedly and this translates into increased surgical survival.

- To date coronary angioplasty has not been proven to prolong life (or shorten it).

Identifying those at risk

The only absolute way to evaluate CAD is by angiography.

Where practical those below 50 years of age should undergo this procedure because decisions made are for 20–30 years and should be based on the fullest possible information. Resources may limit this arbitrary age-level to 40 years.

Electrocardiography

The resting ECG is the most widely applied test in the evaluation of angina pectoris. It is not a substitute for a good clinical history and clinical judgement. It may be normal in up to 50 per cent of patients with angina even in the presence of severe symptoms. A normal ECG therefore does not rule out CAD but it does suggest good left ventricular function. An *abnormal* resting ECG identifies a patient group at higher risk of death and myocardial infarction — changes may be non-specific ST depression or T wave inversion but previous infarction may also be identified. Left bundle branch block suggests left ventricular impairment and possibly multivessel CAD. Old traces should be reviewed if available as changes from normal to abnormal or vice versa may identify ischaemic events new or old.

Exercise testing

An ECG on exercise is safe and accurate. Symptom-limited treadmill exercise testing is of most value. Exercise ECGs are used principally:

- To clarify the chest pain diagnosis — all ages
- To identify those at risk up to 70 years of age
- To objectively assess symptoms and disability
- To monitor progress and assess therapy
- To guide rehabilitation

Medical supervision is essential: the chances of precipitating mortality are 1:10 000, of ventricular fibrillation 1:5000. Full resuscitation must be at hand.

Exercise testing is contraindicated in certain cases:

- Unstable angina
- Significant aortic stenosis
- Pulmonary hypertension
- Severe systemic hypertension
- Known poorly controlled serious ventricular arrhythmias
- Recent myocardial infarct (< 7 days).

The main end-points for a poor prognosis on exercise testing are as follows:

- Significant ST depression >1 mm usually with pain
- Slow ST recovery to normal (5 minutes or greater)
- Fall in systolic blood pressure (reflecting a fall in cardiac output): 20 mmHg or greater
- Rise in diastolic blood pressure (fall in output causes reflex vasoconstriction): >15 mmHg
- Angina with or without ST changes at a low workload: < 6 minutes
- Dangerous arrhythmias — eg, ventricular tachycardia
- ST depression >3 mm without pain.

The ST segment can be modified by digoxin and beta-blockers, which should be discontinued if clinically safe (digoxin 7 days, beta-blockers 48 hours). Nitrates and calcium antagonists should not be taken on the day of the test.

Exercise tests identify low risk in patients:

- Able to exercise to stage 3 or beyond of the Bruce Treadmill protocol with no ST changes

- Who achieve stage 4 or beyond despite ST changes.

Exercise test terminology is as follows:

'True positive':	positive exercise test, proven CAD
'True negative':	negative exercise test, normal coronaries
'False positive':	positive test, normal arteries
'False negative':	negative test, proven CAD
'Sensitivity'(%):	$\dfrac{\text{true +ve}}{\text{true +ves + false -ves}} \times 100$
'Specificity'(%):	$\dfrac{\text{true -ves}}{\text{true -ves + false +ves}} \times 100$
'Predictive accuracy'%:	$\dfrac{\text{true +ve}}{\text{true +ves + false +ves}} \times 100$

Thus 'sensitivity' is the percentage of patients with CAD who have an abnormal exercise ECG, 'specificity' is the percentage of negative tests in patients without CAD and 'predictive accuracy' is the percentage of positive tests that are truly positive.

Thus sensitivity detects patients with disease and specificity excludes those without disease.

- Angina and ST depression >1mm gives a predictive accuracy of 90 per cent for CAD
- ST depression >2 mm is virtually diagnostic for CAD
- ST depression >1 mm and no pain has a predictive value of 70 per cent and >2 mm 90 per cent for CAD
- False positive tests are more common in women
- Overall sensitivity averages 66 per cent and specificity 79 per cent.

Problem areas exist: with left bundle branch block (LBBB), one cannot interpret the ECG; there may be physical limitation (eg, arthritis) or a lack of coordination (so the patient cannot exercise properly).

Ambulatory ECGs

Ambulatory ECGs for 24–48 hours are unhelpful with LBBB but can be of use in evaluating pain when physical limitation prohibits exercise testing, when chest pain occurs at night, or when chest pain is linked to arrhythmias.

Ambulatory monitoring has also identified ST changes in the absence of symptoms — *silent myocardial ischaemia*. This may occur in patients with CAD who never have angina (type 1) or in those who do experience angina but have painful and painless ischaemia (type 2).

Management is controversial but when assessing risk, silent ischaemia on a treadmill ECG does predict an adverse outcome. Ambulatory monitoring is less accurate, however, and should be reserved for selected patients who have proven ischaemic heart disease, eg, previous infarction, and no confusing factors such as LBBB, left ventricular hypertrophy and strain and digoxin therapy.

Nuclear imaging

Nuclear scanning has a limited, but helpful, role in addition to exercise electrocardiography. It needs specialized equipment and is more expensive but is useful in the presence of LBBB, when routine exercise tests are non-diagnostic or borderline, or when cardiovascular stress is limited by poor exercise ability.

Thallium-201 is taken up by the perfused myocardium. Note that:

- Infarction is a 'cold' area which fails to fill in.
- Exercise may cause a cold area which fills in later: this is a sign of reversible ischaemia.
- Partial filling suggests ischaemia adjacent to infarction.

Thallium imaging is superior to exercise testing for the diagnosis of CAD with a sensitivity of 84 per cent versus 66 per cent and specificity of 87 per cent versus 79 per cent. In some studies it has been shown to predict subsequent cardiac events and prognosis more accurately, with event rates related exponentially and independently to both the extent and severity of reversible ischaemia. It is, however, more expensive and requires specialized equipment and the more accurate tomographic techniques (SPECT) are technically demanding — its role remains valuable but limited. It can be helpful in relating the coronary anatomy to the extent of ischaemia when planning angioplasty or CABG. A *normal* thallium scan has a very low event rate — less than 1 per cent — and can be regarded as very reassuring, particularly in the presence of atypical chest pain and equivocal exercise ECGs.

The development of low cost, low radiation, generator produced and easily available radiopharmaceuticals (eg, ^{99m}Tc-sestamibi) offers better imaging than and offers advantages over thallium, as it needs less specialized facilities (ie wider applicability) and there is evidence that SPECT sestamibi (ie, 3-dimensional views) reduces the false-positive rate and improves the specificity for the detection of CAD.

However, while myocardial perfusion imagery is the most important aspect of nuclear cardiology, particularly SPECT, cost will limit its applicability. For the present it is helpful:

- When there is LBBB
- When the functional significance of the established CAD is uncertain
- When exercise stress is not possible, eg, peripheral vascular disease, arthritis
- When the exercise ECG is equivocal
- When ischaemic LV dysfunction is present and the degree of reversibility is questioned
- To assess the success of CABG/PTCA, particularly if atypical symptoms persist.

Those who cannot exercise may have ischaemia induced by dipyridamole.

Positron emission tomography (PET)

This technique uses as tracers positron emitters which have very short half-lives requiring an on-site cyclotron for production and radiochemistry facilities. The technique involves radiation, is expensive and slow but does allow the opportunity for accurate measurement of regional blood flow. In clinical practice it can identify hibernating myocardium in patients where prognosis would be improved by intervention and improved ventricular function. The advantage over thallium is at best marginal and unlikely to justify anything other than highly selected and research use.

Echocardiography

Echocardiography is useful for the non-invasive assessment of LV (its principal use) and valvar function but not of CAD. Echocardiography on exercise may identify ischaemia-induced LV dysfunction. It may be of particular use in women with non diagnostic exercise ECGs.

Technical difficulties in obtaining good images during exercise are circumvented by using pharmacological stressers such as dipyridamole and more recently dobutamine, which looks to be superior. Echos are cheap, safe and reproducible and repeatable and may therefore be of more clinical benefit than radionuclide studies. The place of stress echocardiography is similar to that of nuclear studies as detailed above — it is employed :

- When there is LBBB
- When conventional exercise is not possible
- To assess the degree of ischaemic LV dysfunction
- To assess the functional significance of documented CAD in LV performance
- To judge the value of intervention.

Coronary angiography

Coronary angiography is the best diagnostic test: it accurately assesses the anatomy. A stenosis is significant when the lumen is narrowed by 70 per cent or more or 50 per cent in the left main coronary artery.

Day-case procedures are increasingly employed. Important complications occur in just under 1 per cent, with death in 0.11 per cent. These figures include high-risk cases so routine procedures will be at lower risk.

Coronary anatomy is shown in Figure 8.

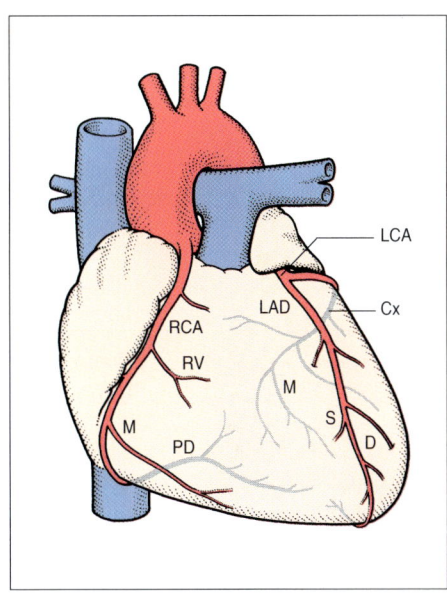

Figure 8
Schematic chart of the major coronary arteries. The posterior descending (PD) may arise from the right coronary artery (RCA; R dominant) or circumflex (Cx; L dominant). D: diagonal; LAD: left anterior descending; LCA: left coronary artery; M: marginal branches; RV: branch to the right ventricle; S: septal branch.

Indications for coronary angiography include symptoms interfering with the quality of life; biological age, not chronological age (so it is applicable to those in their 80s in good health); an abnormal exercise ECG independent of symptoms; and all under 50 years of age with angina — the prognosis reflects CAD extent and LV function.

In Figure 9 I have summarized the investigative approach. This is equivalent to 3 000 exercise tests and 700–1000 angiograms per million of the population per year. A problem group exists and this relates to screening. Here we are dealing with asymptomatic people who are having an 'executive check-up' and those who are worried about CAD because of a family history.

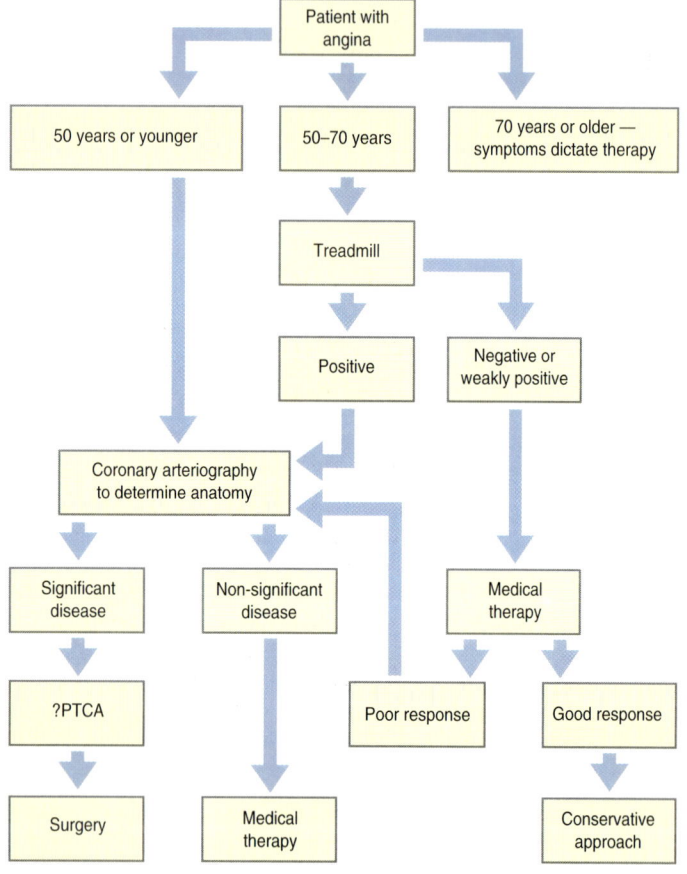

Figure 9
Investigative approach to the clinical evaluation of the patient with angina pectoris. Nuclear imaging and stress echocardiography complement this algorithm in selected cases.

Screening

Lipids It is now clear that in the presence of established CAD, correcting lipid abnormalities reduces disease progression and induces disease regression. The benefits are particularly clear in patients post CABG and, by extrapolation, PTCA. There is no argument that as a part of secondary prevention all patients should undergo full lipid screening up to 80 years of age, with measurements of total, LDL and HDL cholesterol, as well as triglycerides. Whilst it is debatable that the elderly need intervention, they can still be used as a means of identifying younger family members who may be at risk and benefit from primary prevention.

Lipid screening is indicated:

- In all with established CAD to reduce subsequent ischaemic events
- In families of those with familial hypercholesterolaemia
- In other at risk groups, eg, diabetics, hypertensives and those with a strong family history of CAD as both primary and secondary prevention
- *Now* — it is time to get on with it and stop arguing.

Exercise ECGs In the asymptomatic, ECGs are unreliable on exercise (66 per cent false positives). They are, however, useful in those at high risk, eg, familial hypercholesterolaemia (2 per cent of the total population), when an annual review may identify developing CAD.

Otherwise, they are only of value if we are looking for left main stem disease. As this represents only 8 per cent of the angina population, the value of screening the pain-free is extremely limited.

In the UK the Civil Aviation Authority has rejected exercise ECGs for asymptomatic pilots.

Blood pressure A check on blood pressure remains the most useful annual check an asymptomatic person can have.

Silent ischaemia Evaluation has been discussed under ambulatory monitoring (see page 26). Detecting silent ischaemia on exercise testing is a more reliable predictor of CAD than ambulatory monitoring. Thus, the development of silent ischaemia during exercise test screening of those who are asymptomatic but at high risk (eg hypercholesterolaemics) merits angiography. A high incidence of NCA remains.

Management

General management
Drug therapy
Coronary angioplasty
Coronary surgery
Secondary prevention
Coronary disease in women

General management

The management of angina must take into account both the quality and 'quantity' of life. We need to make people not only feel better but also live longer.

In general

There is no substitute for a careful clear explanation of the nature of the problem, the reasons it occurred and how the patient can help himself or herself. The emphasis should be on a team approach, with the patient the most important part of the team. Booklets provide useful repetitive information, answering questions not raised at interview, but although they should be used routinely they are not a substitute for personal contact.

- Smoking: this should be stopped. It may be best to work to a compromise of 5 cigarettes a day and then wean off.
- Obesity: weight loss may reduce anginal frequency.
- Alcohol in moderation is usually beneficial but check lipid status and potential for drug interactions. Alcohol unfortunately is a cause of weight gain and poor diabetic control.
- Exercise: may improve well-being. Though not statistically significant, pooling of studies shows a favourable trend towards a reduction in cardiac events. Avoid isometrics and encourage dynamics (eg, brisk walking, swimming, golf).
- Vigorous exercise (eg, skiing): only if treadmill ECG satisfactory.
- Driving (ordinary): if angina occurs on driving this should be stopped and the licensing authority notified. Otherwise driving is permitted, but advise patients to check their personal insurance status.

- Driving (heavy goods vehicle/public service vehicle): advise against holding a licence even if there is only mild angina. This applies to ambulance, fire, police, taxi and hire-car drivers also. If there is diagnostic doubt a treadmill ECG is essential as a livelihood is at stake.
- Stress: makes other factors worse. Look at lifestyle, workload, leisure time.
- Sex: activity is equal to climbing two flights of stairs (13 steps) briskly. Patients may be helped by GTN beforehand. Extramarital sex is more risky. The rules apply to both homosexuals and heterosexuals.
- Work: 90 per cent can maintain employment but heavy labouring jobs will need to be changed. Stress, hours etc remain important.

Lipids

Hyperlipidaemia is common, with over half of men in the UK having a cholesterol level of 6.5 mmol/l or greater. Familial hypercholesterolaemia (FH) affects 2 per cent of the population and is associated with a significantly increased risk of CAD.

In the presence of established CAD, in this case the patient with angina, all patients should undergo full lipid profile analysis. Whilst HDL is protective, LDL is clearly associated with CAD development (Figure 10). Lowering LDL cholesterol and elevating HDL leads to a reduction in progression of CAD and increases regression of CAD. This is particularly important in CABG patients as the late vein graft failure rate (50 per cent at 10 years) is due to atherosclerosis and can be significantly reduced by lipid lowering therapy.

Table 6 shows the guidelines for introducing lipid lowering drug therapy.

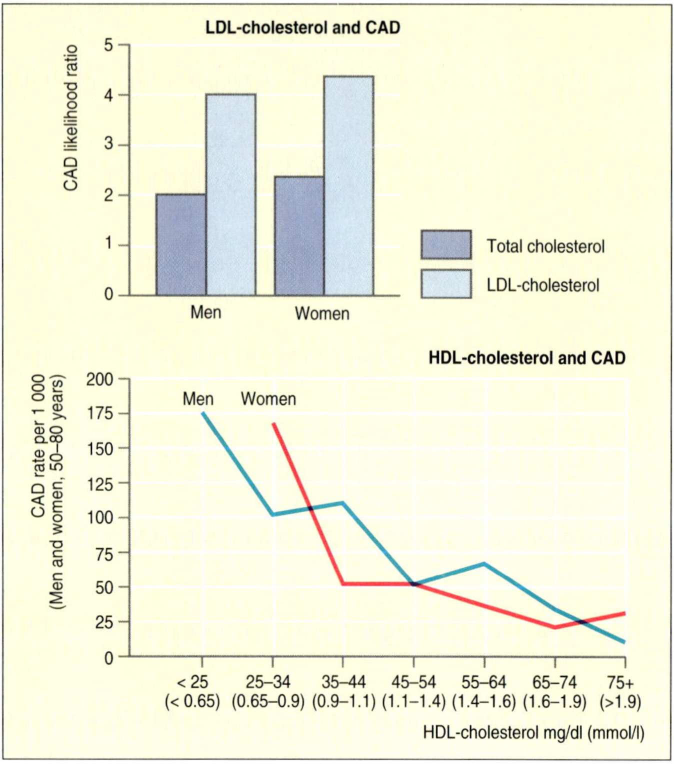

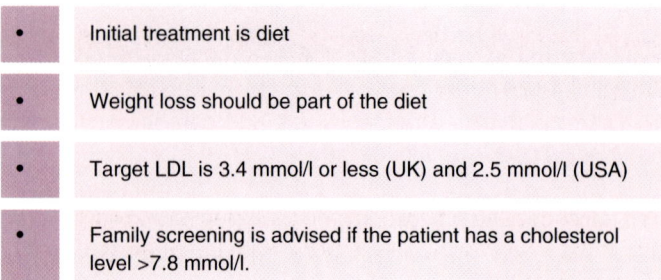

Figure 10
Top: there is a stronger correlation between LDL and CAD than with total cholesterol. Bottom: HDL is a protective factor.

- Initial treatment is diet

- Weight loss should be part of the diet

- Target LDL is 3.4 mmol/l or less (UK) and 2.5 mmol/l (USA)

- Family screening is advised if the patient has a cholesterol level >7.8 mmol/l.

Patient category	Level in mmol/l (mg/dl)	
	Cholesterol	LDL cholesterol
Established CAD, including previous myocardial infarction, angina of effort, post-CABG, angioplasty or cardiac transplant, or other significant atherosclerosis	>5.2 (>200)	>3.4 (>130)
Genetically determined hyperlipidaemia (eg, familial hypercholesterolaemia) or multiple risk factors (adverse family history, diabetes mellitus, hypertension, long smoking history, concomittant raised triglycerides and low HDL cholesterol)	>6.5 (>250)	>5.2 (>200)
Males without evidence of atherosclerosis or other risk factors	>7.8 (>300)	>6.0 (>240)
Post-menopausal females without evidence of other risk factors (ensure raised cholesterol not due to high HDL cholesterol). Take account of premature menopause or too low HDL cholesterol; discuss HRT before considering lipid-lowering medication	>7.8 (>300)	>6.0 (>240)

Table 6
*Cut-off values above which lipid-lowering drug therapy may be of benefit.
Reproduced with permission from Durrington P.* Preventive Cardiology. *London:
Martin Dunitz, 1993.*

The more detailed management of hyperlipidaemia is to be
found in *Preventive Cardiology* by Paul Durrington (London:
Martin Dunitz, 1993).

As a cardiologist I adopt the following practical approach when hyperlipidaemia is present in spite of lifestyle changes (diet, exercise):

- Aim for LDL 3.4 mmol/l or less.
- If second time CABG — 2.5 mmol/l.
- Employ statins (fluvastatin 20–80 mg, pravastatin 10–40 mg and simvastatin 10–40 mg daily); expect a 30 per cent reduction in cholesterol and 15 per cent in triglycerides.
- If triglycerides are a significant problem (>4.0 mmol/l) use fibrates (eg fenofibrate or ciprofibrate); over 30 per cent reduction in triglycerides is likely but the cholesterol reduction is variable, averaging 15–30 per cent.
- Statins and fibrates in combination are very effective but statin-induced myositis incidence is increased. Fluvastatin may avoid this.
- Resistant cases respond to combinations of resins (colestipol and cholestyramine) plus statins plus fibrates.
- Monitor liver function on statins; check for headaches and sleep disturbance on simvastatin.
- Always check for side-effects, particularly with resins.

Most patients respond to a statin and diet with both statins and fibrates being well tolerated. It is important not to compromise too soon. It is always necessary to look for secondary causes, in particular, hypothyroidism, diabetes and excess alcohol intake. It is essential to know not only the total cholesterol but also the HDL and LDL, particularly in women who may have high HDLs which are protective and should not be reduced.

Drug therapy

There are three classes of drugs used for the treatment of stable angina:

- Nitrates

- Beta-blockers

- Calcium antagonists.

Nitrates

Nitrates are potent venodilators and to a lesser extent arterial dilators (Table 7). They act by reducing demand, and the main benefit is from peripheral vasodilatation.

They are safe in combination with calcium antagonists and beta-blockers; and are safe when LV function is impaired.

Sublingual

Sublingual nitrates avoid hepatic metabolism.

They are effective in 1–2 minutes (the spray is quicker than the tablets), and the effect lasts 30 minutes. The tablets lose potency over two months and should be stored in a cool place in a dark glass bottle without cotton-wool; the spray shelf-life is three years.

Sublingual nitrates may be used for angina relief and prophylactically. Headache is the main side-effect — the patient should be warned. Syncope is rare, but more common in the elderly when standing.

All patients should be prescribed and instructed on the use of sublingual nitrates. Most patients prefer the spray, although it is more expensive.

Preparation	Use	Comments
Sublingual GTN 500 µg	Alleviates attacks quickly; prophylaxis 30 minutes	Headaches. Replenish every 2 months. Careful storage
GTN spray 400 µg	Alleviates attacks quickly; prophylaxis 30 minutes	Expensive. Headaches. Inflammable
Topical nitrates	Nocturnal symptoms? Debatable whether they are useful	Expensive, short duration of action, patch cosmetically better than paste.
Isosorbide dinitrate 1 sublingual 2 oral	Prophylaxis 1 hour Prevention of pain. 10–40 mg bid	As GTN. Hepatic metabolism ↑ Tolerance ↑ if tds or qds
Isosorbide mononitrate	Prevention of pain. 10–40 mg bid	100 per cent bioavailability. Preferable to dinitrate.
Buccal nitrates	Alleviate pain and prophylaxis	Expensive, variably tolerated. Useful when oral therapy not possible.

Table 7
Nitrate preparations

Buccal nitrates

Buccal nitrates combine immediate nitrate release with a gradual release over four hours. They are effective agents but there is variable patient acceptability. Dosage is 1, 2, 3 or 5 mg. They are expensive. They are useful when oral therapy is not possible (eg, pre- or post-operation), and can be beneficial in severe cases with nocturnal symptoms. Their rapid disappearance tends to avoid tolerance.

Oral

The active metabolite mononitrate is now available in pure form with 100 per cent bioavailability. The dinitrate relies on hepatic metabolism for conversion to the mononitrate, leading to substantial variability between and within patients.

Oral mononitrate is recommended. Nitrate tolerance (defined as decreasing effect with time) is a problem and is caused by consistent exposure to nitrates resulting in vascular tolerance. Tolerance can be prevented by avoiding consistent high concentrations and allowing low nitrate or nitrate-free periods.

- Conventional mononitrate can be titrated from 10 mg bid to 20 and then 40 mg bid
- Allow 12 hours between doses or use asymmetical dosing, eg 8am and 2pm
- Most benefit is at 20 mg bid
- Once-daily preparations are a convenient alternative as 25 mg, 40 mg, 50 mg or 60 mg preparations — reducing tolerance and increasing compliance.

Mononitrates can be co-prescribed safely with both calcium antagonists and beta-blockers to obtain additive effects.

Topical nitrates

Topical nitrates avoid hepatic metabolism, but consistent blood levels lead to rapid tolerance. Intermittent use (12 hours on, 12 off) is effective but expensive. Dosage is 5, 10 or 15 mg.

Because topical nitrates require nitrate-free periods to be effective they cannot be used safely as monotherapy.

They may help nocturnal pain (when put on at night, and taken off in the morning). The location of the patch is not important, but there is psychological benefit if it is put on the chest.

Nitrate side-effects

Side-effects are headache; syncope (alcohol may enhance this); tachycardia (not frequent); rarely, methaemoglobinaemia in a high dose; facial flushing; and halitosis (with sublingual tablets). Nitrates are contraindicated in hypertrophic obstructive cardiomyopathy — a rare cause of angina.

Beta-blockade

Beta-adrenergic blockade reduces sympathetically mediated effects on myocardial demand by reducing heart rate, reducing blood pressure and reducing contractility.

The action is competitive, and leads to a reduction in anginal attacks and the need for GTN, as well as leading to an increase in exercise ability with less ischaemia on the ECG. Ischaemic episodes over 24 hours, whether painful or silent, are reduced.

Beta-blockade is effective in over 90 per cent of patients.

Cardioselective beta-blockade

There is preferential action at β_1 receptors in the heart; β_2 receptors are more prominent in the lung and blood vessels (the difference is relative, not absolute).

Cardioselectivity decreases with increasing dose (ie, atenolol 100 mg is less selective than 50 mg). Non-selective and selective agents similarly depress cardiac output, so peripheral side-effects are often similar.

Partial agonist activity

Partial agonist activity (PAA) is also known as 'intrinsic sympathomimetic activity' (ISA).

At low levels of activity it may stimulate beta-receptors rather than block them. Heart rate may be little affected at rest or asleep, but is reduced on exercise, as for agents without PAA. It is likely to be less effective in severe angina when the resting rate needs reduction. It is likely to have fewer peripheral adverse effects because it depresses cardiac output less (eg, less cold hands and feet).

PAA increases with increasing dose to a plateau earlier than agents without PAA, so the total equivalent blockade may not be reached.

Using beta-blockers
The reason for first-line use of beta-blockers is more scientifically established than it is for any other agent in use.

- Prognostically, post infarction there is benefit for agents without PAA

- Infarcts occurring on beta-blockade are smaller

- The influence of sudden stress/shock is reduced

- They are effective across all ages and groups, including smokers and non-smokers.

The most effective means of monitoring effective dosage is by using drugs you are familiar with. The resting heart rate alone is a simple guide to beta-blockade but it is the exercise heart rate that determines full effectiveness. A resting rate of 50 bpm is not an indication for dose reduction unless there are symptoms such as excessive lethargy or effort fatigue.

Guideline optimal levels are atenolol 100 mg daily, propranolol 80 mg tds or dose equivalents. Individuals should be titrated to effect (eg, atenolol 50 mg daily increasing to 100 mg or rarely 200 mg daily).

Adverse effects
The adverse effects are largely predictable and often caused by inappropriate patient selection. It is not logical to use even car-

dioselective beta-blockers in a patient with bronchospasm without using nitrates and calcium antagonists as a safer initial option.

- Bronchoconstriction: these are β_2 effects.
- Heart failure: beta-blockade may significantly reduce output when LV impaired.
- Masking hypoglycaemia: beta-blockade blunts tachycardia.
- Peripheral effects: these include cold hands and feet, heavy legs, aching muscles. These are due to reduced output, not to selectivity, and are less likely with PAA property.
- Central nervous system effects: these include muzzy head, loss of memory, poor concentration, vivid dreams. They are more common with lipid-soluble agents (lipophilic) which cross blood–brain barrier, than with water-soluble (hydrophilic) agents.
- Impotence: this is probably related to the cardiac output reduction. It may affect 10 per cent: it is often under-reported, but should be routinely asked about ('Some of my patients have noticed sexual problems on these drugs — have you noticed anything?').
- Lipids: the effects are much debated. Changes are variable and not on a large scale; they are less likely with selective agents and agents with PAA. There is mainly a reduction in high-density lipoprotein (HDL) cholesterol and elevation of triglycerides; these do not outweigh the proven advantages of beta-blockade.

Beta-blockers available

There is a plethora of agents, summarized in Table 8. The following points represent my personal preferences. Use agents that are cardioselective, hydrophilic, once or twice daily. Stick to one or two drugs and use them optimally.

Atenolol is my preferred agent: it is cardioselective and hydrophilic, and works once daily at 50, 100 and 200 mg, but twice daily at 25 mg dosage. Peak blood levels occur 3–4

Table 8
Beta-blockers available.

Note How to use this table: Assume propanolol as the reference drug with a potency of 1. Propranolol 80 mg can be given twice daily (half-life 11 hours). It is equal to atenolol 100 mg (potency 1:1) and atenolol can be given once daily (pharmacodynamic half-life 24 hours). Sotalol is one-third the potency of propranolol so that it needs to be given 240 mg once daily to be equivalent to propranolol 80 mg bid, ie, we compare dosage with 80 mg propranolol equivalent, not with total daily dose.

Drug	Potency	Cardio-selective	Optimum dose dynamic half-life hours	Blood–brain barrier penetration	Dosage adjust-ments
Acebutolol	0.3[a]	+[b]	24	NS	Renal
Atenolol	1	+	24	NS	Renal
Bisoprolol	10	+	24	Yes	None
Metoprolol	1	+	10–12	Yes	Liver
Nadolol	1.5	0	39	NS	Renal
Oxprenolol	0.5–1[a]	0	13	Yes	Liver
Pindolol	6[a]	0	8	Yes	None
Propranolol	1	0	11	Yes++	Liver
Sotalol	0.3	0	24	NS	Renal
Timolol	6	0	15	Yes	Liver
Slow oxprenolol	[a]		< 24		
Metoprolol SA			24		
Propranolol LA			24		

[a] *Agents with PAA (ISA).* [b] *Cardioselectivity of acebutolol is debated. NS, not significant.*

hours post dose and correlate with fatigue side-effects. Therefore it is often prescribed for the evening. Begin at 25 mg in the elderly and 50 mg in those below 70 years.

Propranolol is highly lipophilic and to be used principally when there is a high level of anxiety. The dose is 40 mg tds, 80 mg bid or tds or l60 mg bid.

Acebutolol is cardioselective and hydrophilic with PAA. It is a twice- or once-daily agent depending on dose. Use it when peripheral adverse effects are a problem or likely to be so (eg, with coexisting claudication). It is not as effective in severe cases as the resting rate is not suppressed to the same degree. The dose is 100 mg bid, 200 mg bid and 400 mg once or twice daily.

All patients with stable angina should be considered for beta-blockade at the same time as sublingual nitrates are prescribed.

Beta-blockers should not be suddenly withdrawn from therapy as rebound effects can occur, leading to unstable angina or infarction. This is less of a problem with long-acting agents such as atenolol or less potent agents with PAA.

Beta-blockers all share the same mechanism of action — competition at the beta-receptor — so full effect depends on optimal dosage.

Calcium antagonists

Since they were first introduced in the 1960s these drugs have proven to be effective in the management of chronic stable angina and hypertension but they unfortunately lack any significant prognostic benefits post myocardial infarction. They do not protect the patient from abrupt withdrawal of beta-blockade.

Calcium ions are essential for myocardial contraction and conduction. Calcium antagonists act by impairing the influx of these ions into smooth muscle, myocardial and conducting tissue cells. The effects can be summarized: myocardial contractility may be reduced; conduction may be depressed; and coronary and peripheral vascular tone is relaxed.

Different calcium antagonists have different properties and these variations are extremely important — much more important than the differences between the beta-blockers (Table 9).

Effect on	Amlodipine	Nicardipine	Nifedipine	Verapamil	Diltiazem
Heart rate	0(↑)	↑	↑	0↓	0↓
Atrioventricular conduction	0	0	0	↓↓	↓
Peripheral vasodilation	+++	+++	+++	++	++
Coronary vasodilation	+++	+++	+++	++	++
Contractility	0(↓)	↓0	↓0	↓↓	↓

Table 9
The calcium antagonists. Amlodipine has minimal effects on heart rate and contractility.

Verapamil and diltiazem may reduce heart rate, atrioventricular conduction and cardiac output. Diltiazem has more effect on the sino-atrial node than verapamil but less effect on atrioventricular (AV) conduction and cardiac output. Both have modest peripheral dilating effects, diltiazem more than verapamil. The dihydropyridine calcium-channel antagonists (amlodipine, felodipine, isradipine, lacidipine, nicardipine and nifedipine) are principally peripheral and coronary vasodilators. They are less likely to depress cardiac output because any deleterious effects are offset by afterload reduction due to peripheral vasodilation. Caution is strongly advised in the presence of significant LV dysfunction, however, particularly if combined with beta-blockade. They have no effect on cardiac conduction. Currently approved for angina are amlodipine, nifedipine and nicardipine. Felodipine, lacidipine and isradipine are only approved for hypertension at the present time.

Using calcium antagonists

Calcium antagonists have gained widespread acceptance for the treatment of anginal patients because of their proven efficacy and their lack of the fatiguing side-effects that unfortunately limit beta-blockade. In addition, their vasodilating properties may be beneficial in Raynaud's phenomenon and when bronchospasm is a problem. Verapamil and diltiazem may be useful in non-Q wave infarction and prevention of re-infarction, providing left ventricular function is good, but, overall, calcium antagonists are of little or no value in the immediate post-myocardial infarction patient and in this situation should be considered only for those intolerant of beta-blockade or when beta-blockade is contraindicated. Considerable interest has been generated concerning the potential beneficial effects on atheroma progression and regression in humans (INTACT)* but this needs translating into clinical benefit also.

In general calcium antagonists can be advocated:

- As an alternative to beta-blockade

- When beta-blockers are contraindicated

- When beta-blockers induce adverse effects

- In addition to nitrates

- In addition to beta-blockers, but only dihydropyridines are totally safe because a conduction interaction is absent. Verapamil should be avoided and diltiazem used very carefully

- When bronchospasm is also present because of potentially beneficial actions on bronchial smooth muscle tone as well as angina.

* Lichtlen PR, Hugenholtz PG, Rafflenbeul W et al. Retardation of angiographic pro-gression of coronary artery disease by nifedipine (INTACT). Lancet (1990) **335**:1109–13.

Verapamil is a powerful antiarrhythmic drug particularly suitable for supraventricular tachycardias. It has comparable efficacy to beta-blockade as monotherapy, but is not safe to co-prescribe with beta-blockade. It is the most cardiac-depressant of the calcium antagonists. There is a significant interaction with digoxin which may affect AV conduction and increase digoxin levels and side-effects. The dosage is 40–160 mg tds. Slow-release formulations are also available and can be used when stable on conventional formulations.

Adverse effects include flushing and headaches secondary to vasodilatation and constipation (especially in the elderly). High-fibre diets may help but constipation can be severe and verapamil must be discontinued. Verapamil rarely impairs liver function. Although it causes fluid retention and vasodilatation side-effects, these are less than with dihydropyridines.

Diltiazem is similar to verapamil but causes less depression of AV conduction and cardiac contraction. It is an effective mono-therapy in angina, equivalent to beta-blockade. It may be used with beta-blockade but is less safe than dihydropyridines: caution is advised on initiation, and it is advisable to co-prescribe only with the patient in hospital because of the bradycardia risks. Co-prescription is effective when coronary spasm is documented.

The adverse effects of diltiazem are as for verapamil but less constipation is reported. Fluid retention may be more of a problem, or be seen more as it is prescribed on a wider basis.

The dosage is 60 mg to 120 mg tds (twice-daily for elderly patients). Slow-release preparations are available but limited information is available regarding their efficacy. Diltiazem is clinically better tolerated than verapamil, and is usually used in preference unless supraventricular arrhythmias feature signifi-cantly in the anginal presentation.

Dihydropyridines include amlodipine, nicardipine and nifedip-ine for angina pectoris. They are potent arterial vasodilators acting by relaxing vascular smooth muscle. There is less effect on myocardial contraction but their use is still unwise if LV func-tion is impaired substantially. They have no antiarrhythmic actions, and are safe with beta-blockade. They are especially effective when coronary spasm is considered a component. However, this is rare (< 5 per cent) in stable angina.

The adverse effects reflect more vasodilatation, therefore it is more likely for there to be flushing, headaches and diuretic-resistant fluid retention (at the ankles and/or abdomen). Eye pain and gum hyperplasia are reported with nifedipine. Occasionally, ischaemic pain can follow the ingestion of nifedipine and nicardipine. This may reflect the drugs' rapid onset of action, a heart rate increase or a coronary steal effect: in such cases therapy must be stopped. The longer acting agent amlodipine provides 24-hour cover and has a more gradual onset of action, minimizing the cardiovascular reflexes which increase heart rate and making it a safer agent as monotherapy. Amlodipine also appears to have fewer negative effects on LV function.

No lipid adverse effects have been reported with calcium antagonists. The drugs are not as effective as beta-blockers in smokers.

Amlodipine is currently the most convenient: it is used once daily, aiding compliance, has a less rapid onset of action and is reportedly more selective for the vasculature or myocardium than nifedipine or nicardipine.

Sorting out the differences
Verapamil and diltiazem should mainly be seen as alternatives to beta-blockade with occasional co-prescribing cautiously with diltiazem. Diltiazem is generally better tolerated but verapamil is more effective if supraventricular arrhythmias occur.

The three currently approved dihydrophyridines are very similar in action. Little difference exists between nifedipine and nicardipine, both of which are equally as effective as nitrates as monotherapy but less effective than beta-blockade.

- Nifedipine is convenient in the retard preparation, 10 mg or 20 mg twice daily. In the elderly begin with 5 mg tds.

- Nicardipine is inconvenient. Dose is 20 mg, increasing to 40 mg tds. No significant advantage in its formulation justifies its use above nifedipine or amlodipine.

- Shorter acting agents (nifedipine, nicardipine and isradipine) are more likely than longer-acting agents (amlodipine) to induce angina due to reflex tachycardia. They should not be used as monotherapy but are safe in combination with beta-blockade.

- Amlodipine is currently the most useful agent: its once-daily effectiveness aids compliance and it appears to have a lower incidence of side-effects. The minimal risk of heart rate increase renders it safe as monotherapy. Dosage is 5 or 10 mg once daily.

Combination therapy

Beta-blockade plus mononitrates are additive. Calcium antagonists plus nitrates are additive. Beta-blockade plus calcium antagonists are additive.

The commonest combination is a beta-blocker plus a calcium antagonist or mononitrate and triple therapy reflects the use of all three agents. Typical are:

- Atenolol 50 or 100 mg plus amlodipine 5 or 10 mg day

- Atenolol 50 mg or 100 mg plus ISMN slow release 40/50/ 60 mg day

- Atenolol plus ISMN plus amlodipine.

When beta-blockers are contraindicated the frequent combinations are:

- Verapamil 40–160 mg tds plus ISMN

- Diltiazem 60–120 mg tds plus ISMN

- Amlodipine 5–10 mg once daily plus ISMN.

Triple therapy induces a variable response and a switch might be better than adding in (Figure 11). However, angina 'needing' triple therapy should be investigated further and angioplasty or surgery considered. An overview is given in Figure 12.

Atenolol plus diltiazem may be effective but runs the risk of conduction and cardiac contraction problems, particularly brady-

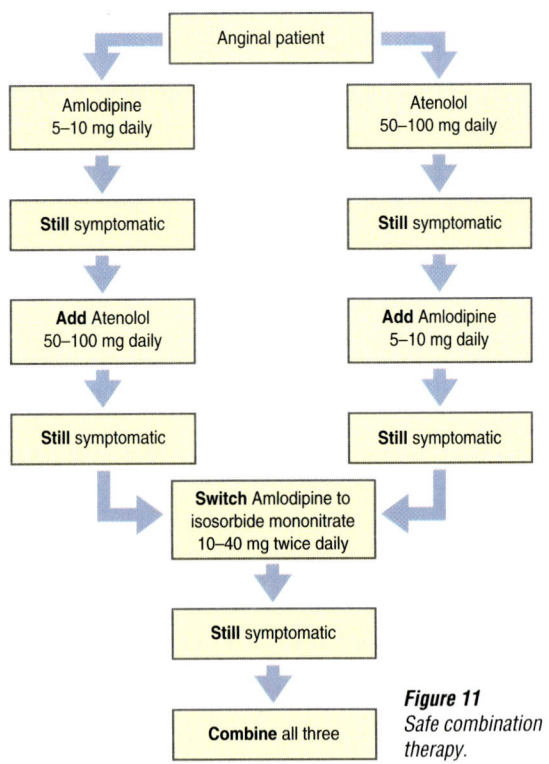

Figure 11
Safe combination therapy.

cardia. It is best initiated at atenolol 50 mg om and diltiazem 60 mg tds to limit the potential for adverse interaction, and dose adjustments can be made subsequently depending on effect.

- Some patients can become worse when the third agent is added to double therapy

- Always use drugs in optimal dosage but consider a combination of two low-dose drugs if side-effects occur, eg atenolol 50 mg plus amlodipine 5 mg rather than atenolol 100 mg alone.

Aspirin

In low doses, aspirin inhibits platelet aggregation, reducing the risk of vascular death, stroke and myocardial infarction by about 25 per cent. Both men and women benefit irrespective of age, diabetes or hypertension. A dose of 75 mg/day minimizes gastrointestinal side-effects and is a highly cost-effective and safe treatment. Active peptic ulceration or known aspirin hypersensitivity are contraindications.

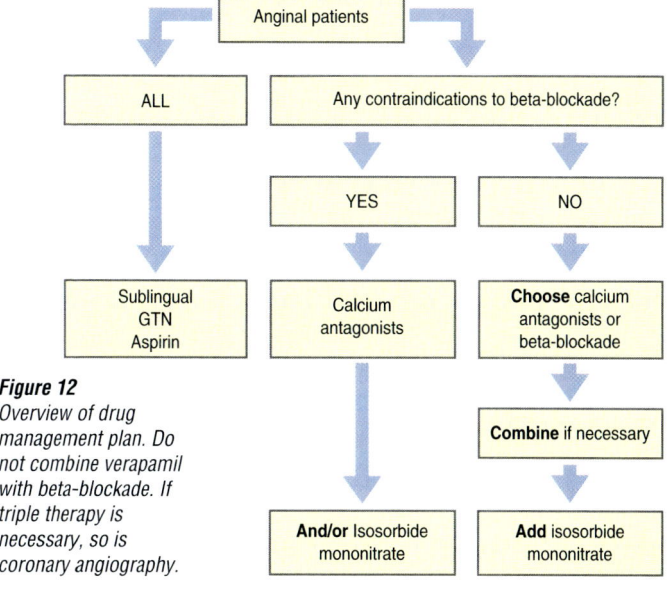

Figure 12
Overview of drug management plan. Do not combine verapamil with beta-blockade. If triple therapy is necessary, so is coronary angiography.

Percutaneous transluminal coronary angioplasty (PTCA) has given the physician for the first time the possibility of increasing the supply of blood to the heart rather than reducing demand (Figure 13).

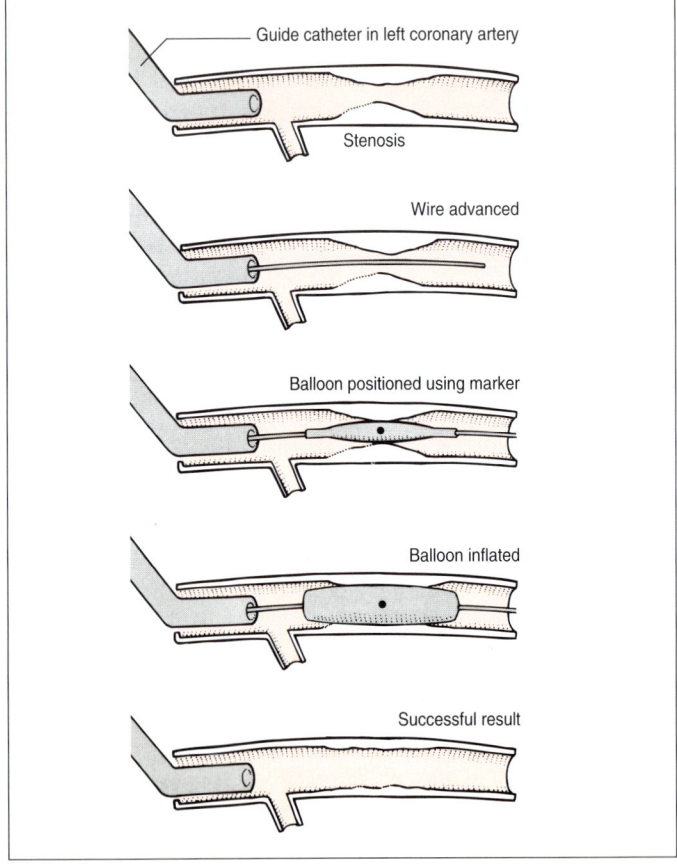

Guide catheter in left coronary artery

Stenosis

Wire advanced

Balloon positioned using marker

Balloon inflated

Successful result

Figure 13
The technique of angioplasty.

The procedure is similar to coronary angiography: the stenosis is identified, a guide-wire passed over it and a balloon advanced along the guide-wire until it crosses the lesion. The balloon is then inflated and hopefully the stenosis substantially reduced.

Who should have PTCA?

The primary indication for PTCA in the patient with angina is the same as for CABG — to relieve pain. Originally used for single-vessel disease, it is now more widely used for multivessel disease — about 20 per cent of cases. PTCA is less invasive than CABG and can be employed in all age groups. It is effective after CABG when new lesions develop in native vessels or grafts.

Patients with unstable angina (see page 70) can be treated with PTCA but the complications are greater than in stable angina.

- Initial success rate depends on case selection but averages 90 per cent
- Non-fatal infarcts occur in 2 per cent
- Abrupt vessel close affects 5 per cent. This can be treated by repeat balloon dilatation or stent insertion but 2 per cent will require emergency CABG
- Death occurs in less than 1 per cent
- Risks increase as the complexity of the case increases and in emergency situations.

Clinical trials

PTCA versus drug therapy*
In a randomized study of 212 patients with single-vessel CAD who had symptoms or exercise ECG evidence of ischaemia, PTCA was compared with conventional medical therapy.

* Parisi AF, Folland ED, Hartigan P on behalf of the Veterans Affairs ACME investigators. A comparison of angioplasty with medical therapy in the treatment of single-vessel coronary artery disease. N Engl J Med (1992) **326**:10–16.

At six months, of the 105 patients allocated to PTCA and the 107 patients allocated to medicine:

- Freedom from angina was present in 64 per cent of the PTCA group versus 46 per cent medical

- Urgent CABG was needed for 2 patients in the PTCA group

- 16 patients needed repeat PTCA

- PTCA patients increased their exercise ability to a greater degree.

Thus PTCA in suitable patients with amenable single lesions is a useful alternative to medical and CABG treatment in those with moderate to severe angina. This does not apply to those with single-vessel disease and mild angina, who may be better treated medically, or those with less favourable lesions, who may have more complications.

PTCA versus CABG

Several trials are now in progress and interim results have been presented. The most comprehensive data are available from the Randomized Intervention Treatment of Angina Trial (RITA-1)*. However, all trials have so far shown similar findings. The RITA results are summarized in Table 10.

Thus, in the RITA trial, CABG involved a longer initial hospitalization and convalescence than PTCA, but during the following 2.5 years, CABG provided greater relief of angina and a lower risk of further therapeutic intervention.

A follow-up analysis of cost in the RITA trial shows that at two years PTCA cost 80 per cent of CABG but the curves are

* RITA trial participants. Coronary angioplasty versus coronary artery bypass surgery: the Randomized Interventional Treatment of Angina (RITA) trial. Lancet (1993) **341**:573–80.

Table 10
The RITA trial compared the long-term results of coronary angioplasty (PTCA)
and coronary bypass surgery (CABG) at 16 UK centres. Reproduced with
permission from Henderson RA. Angina: medical treatment, coronary
arteriography and angioplasty. Medicine International *(1993)* **21 (10)***:389–400.*

The RITA trial

Patients were eligible for the trial if:

- Myocardial revascularization was considered necessary on clinical grounds
- A cardiologist and cardiothoracic surgeon agreed that equivalent revascularization of one, two or three major coronary arteries could be achieved by either PTCA or CABG.

The trial recruited 1011 patients; in this group:

- The median age was 57 years
- 19 per cent were women
- Severe (grade 3 or 4) angina was present in 59 per cent
- 55 per cent had disease in two or more major coronary arteries.

Interim results were reported in 1993 after a mean of 2.5 years' follow-up; they showed that

- The randomized procedure was carried out in 97 per cent
- The median length of hospital stay for the randomized procedure was 12 days for CABG patients but 4 days for PTCA patients
- Emergency CABG was required in 4 per cent of the PTCA group
- The risk of death or myocardial infarction during the treatment and follow-up periods was similar in the two treatment groups
- Over 2 years, 38 per cent of the PTCA group and 11 per cent of the CABG group experienced a major cardiac event (death, myocardial infarction or additional revascularization procedure)
- Both procedures were effective in relieving symptoms — after 6 months, 89 per cent of the CABG group and 68 per cent of the PTCA group were free from angina, but at 2 years this difference was less marked
- Anti-anginal medication was prescribed more widely among the PTCA patients.

closing and it is possible that at five years the costs will be equal. However, they may diverge again after five years as vein graft failure rates increase.

Restenosis

The Achilles heel of PTCA affects 30–40 per cent at six months but may present with a recurrence of symptoms earlier — 3–4 months. Aspirin and heparin immediately after angioplasty reduce the risk of acute closure, with aspirin recommended indefinitely (75 mg/day). The major problem of long-term restenosis has so far not been influenced by any pharmacological therapy.

- Restenosis presents with angina in 70–80 per cent
- Restenosis is asymptomatic in 10–20 per cent
- Restenosis is more common in the proximal left anterior descending artery, total occlusions (chronic), osteal lesions, long lesions, in the proximal and middle section of vein grafts
- Patients more at risk of restenosis are: male, smokers, diabetics, those unstable at the procedure.

One definition of restenosis is a lesion of greater than 50 per cent at follow-up angiography. More precise definitions using quantitative angiography are used for research studies.

Repeat dilatation is often as successful as the initial procedure with a similar restenosis rate up to five or six attempts.

Stents

These are metallic 'cages' which expand to compress the stenosis. They are delivered on a balloon which is inflated to expand the stent in the correct position. They have been used when the vessel abruptly closes at the time of PTCA or to stabilize severe post-PTCA dissections. Of particular interest is their role in reducing restenosis.

The Benestent trial compared PTCA with elective stenting; 257 patients underwent PTCA and 259 had stents inserted. The results are shown in Table 11.

Results of the Benestent trial*		
	PTCA	**STENT**
Bleeding complications (%)	3.1	13.5
Hospital stay (days)	3	8.5
Repeat PTCA (n)	53	26 } significant
Restenosis (n)	32	22

Table 11
* Awaiting publication.

Stents therefore reduce restenosis when electively implanted but have more complications and a longer hospital stay. The bleeding problems from arterial access reflect the anticoagulant regime needed to prevent thrombosis within the stent. This is likely to be simplified. Also hospital stay is now averaging two days for PTCA and five days for stents. Current advice is warfarin for 2 months after a stent but this may change. To reduce thrombotic complications, stents of 3 mm or more are recommended.

- Stents are considered to be significantly superior to PTCA for vein graft lesions

- All stents are made differently and results for one are not necessarily applicable to others.

Other devices

Atherectomy which is a device for removing atheroma has not been shown to improve on PTCA results and is associated with a similar restenosis rate but greater complications and a disturbing increase in late deaths has been reported.

Lasers have demonstrated no advantages and the rotational device for opening tough lesions has a high complication and restenosis rate.

Atherectomy and rotational devices are likely to have better defined but limited uses in the future.

To summarize

Though we do not yet know whether prognostically PTCA is the same as CABG (or better or worse) we do know that it relieves symptoms, and in 7 out of 10 the benefit is maintained to 6 months. Once the 6-month hurdle is overcome long-term follow-up is encouraging, with 80 per cent free from cardiac events and 70 per cent symptom-free at 4 years.

In clinical practice PTCA should be considered:

- If symptomatic on therapy and the lesions are suitable in one, two or three vessels

- If minimal symptoms but a strongly positive exercise test and appropriate lesions

- If the results at the centre are good enough

- At all times the risk/benefit ratio for the individual patient must be calculated

- Surgical back-up is in my view essential, even though little used now. Avoidable deaths should be avoided

- The operators must undergo comprehensive training — casual angioplasters are dangerous

- Stents are preferable in vein grafts and when there is an abrupt closure or severe dissection

- Restenosis remains a major problem. Primary stenting in larger vessels (>3 mm) may reduce this significantly.

Coronary surgery

The role of CABG in stable angina for relief of symptoms and to lengthen life is well established (see page 20). It is effective in all age-groups, and those over 70 years who are otherwise fit benefit as well as younger patients.

Operative mortality is < 2 per cent under 70 years but may rise to 5 per cent in the elderly and for complex and/or repeat procedures. Graft patency at 12 months is 85–90 per cent on aspirin alone. There is no advantage in using dipyridamole. At 10 years the internal mammary grafts are 95 per cent successful but only 50 per cent of veins are in satisfactory condition.

Surgery is the preferred option over PTCA when total occlusions are present and are believed to be older than 3 months.

In the section on PTCA the merits of PTCA and CABG have been discussed. In Figure 14 the major PTCA-versus-bypass trials are summarized. Surgery leads to a more complete revascularization and a reduced intervention rate. PTCA is a less traumatic procedure with less hospital stay and a more rapid return to normal activities. PTCA and CABG are, however, complimentary. PTCA may delay or prevent the need for CABG and may deal with recurrent problems after CABG.

Morbidity

The aftercare is helped by a full and detailed explanation in the pre-operative period, reinforced by booklets and videos.

Problems encountered include sternum, back and leg pain with muscular pain often recurring over 2–3 months (analgesia and anti-inflammatory agents may be necessary). Neurological problems have been reported in 5–6 per cent, with visual disturbances in up to 20 per cent. However, major residual disability affects only 1–2 per cent. Psychiatric morbidity is related to pre-operative psychiatric and social maladjustment, neurotic personality traits and a previous history of psychiatric illness, and not to the operation itself. Previous peptic ulceration may be exacerbated, and ranitidine is used for peri-operative protection.

Following cardiac surgery, a period of 2–3 months to recover and rehabilitate is strongly advised. Return to work is possible in three months and driving a motor car at one month (though heavy front-wheel drive may give chest wall pain). For heavy goods vehicle/public service vehicle licences a detailed evaluation will be needed at six months.

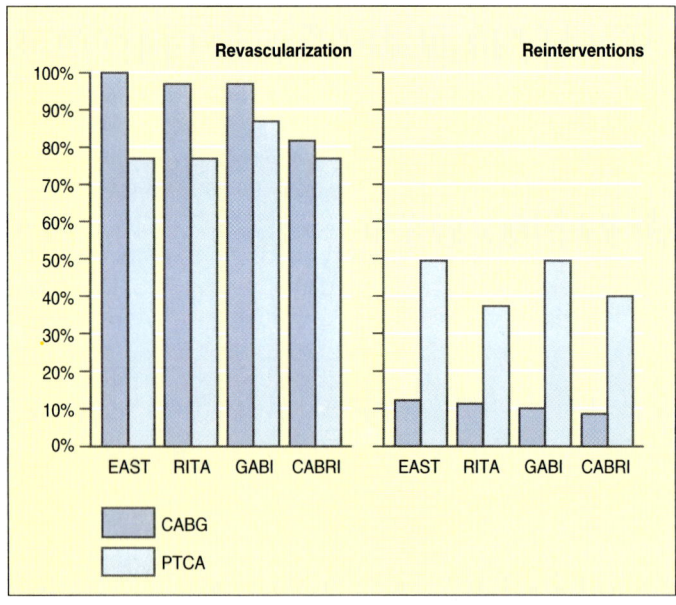

Figure 14
The four major trials comparing PTCA with CABG: CABG affords more complete revascularization and less reintervention subsequently. Derived from PTCA *(1994)* **9/1**.

A rehabilitation programme is strongly recommended after bypass surgery, promoting confidence, exercise ability and affording the opportunity for communication and discussion of problems and objectives.

CABG should be undertaken:

- When symptoms are refractory to medical therapy

- When the anatomy dictates a poor prognosis otherwise

- When PTCA is unsuccessful

- When PTCA is not possible.

Specific points

- 1-year survival after CABG is 95 per cent
- 10-year survival is 80 per cent in non-smokers and 69 per cent in those who continue to smoke
- 80 per cent are free of symptoms up to 5 years and 50 per cent for 10 years. This may improve with wider use of arterial grafts, particularly the left internal mammary artery, and greater attention to lipids
- Abnormal lipids are a major risk for atheroma development and new lesions are reduced to 14 per cent in native vessels and 16 per cent in vein grafts if lipid levels are vigorously reduced by drugs, versus 40 per cent and 35 per cent respectively when treated by diet alone
- Many drugs are inadvertently stopped at surgery and review of lipid profiles and hypertensive care is essential.

Secondary prevention

Most of the studies relate to infarction rather than angina. However, several areas are clear.

Lipids

It is important to measure the lipid profile principally to exclude familial hypercholesterolaemia. Family screening follows from FH detection.

Many people with angina are overweight, and reducing weight and animal fats will be beneficial not only to the lipid profile but also to symptoms, mobility and well-being. Hyperlipidaemia not responding to at least three months' diet should be treated with drugs:

- After CABG — because of clear evidence that native and graft atheroma benefits

- After PTCA — extrapolating mainly from CABG data

- If the LDL cholesterol remains raised above 3.4 mmol/l given that the presence of CAD is proven.

Target total cholesterol is 5.2 mmol/l (200 mg) or less. Efforts should be made to reduce LDL below 3.4 mmol/l (130 mg) and as close to 2.5 mmol/l (96 mg) as possible (see page 35).

Other factors

Smoking
Smoking must be stopped or reduced to three or four cigarettes a day. A compromise often aids compliance, enabling further reduction later. Non-inhaled pipe or cigar smoking is a safer option.

Aspirin
Aspirin can be recommended at 75 mg/day.

Exercise training
Exercise training is recommended for the psychological and physical benefit from feeling fit: it need not be obsessional and must be enjoyed. Regular brisk walking, cycling, swimming etc should be encouraged. There is also a possible prognostic benefit.

Hypertension
Hypertension needs therapy with agents aimed also at angina relief (eg, beta-blockers and calcium antagonists).

Stress
Stress supplements other factors rather like a trigger on a gun. Lifestyle changes should be looked at and in severe cases stress counselling will be beneficial. Stress is an individual perception of life and advice needs to be individualized.

Coronary disease in women

Coronary artery disease is the commonest cause of death for women. Approximately five times as many women die of CAD than breast cancer. Though less frequent under the age of 65 years, it is a diagnosis which should always be considered in the presence of chest pain. Women with CAD present with angina more frequently than myocardial infarction, but their pain is often atypical and difficult to pin down. Exercise tests are more often false positive for CAD especially in young women who have a low incidence of CAD. Over the age of 65 years, exercise tests are more accurate reflecting the increased incidence of CAD in the older female population (about 1 in 3).

Women with CAD are more frequently diabetic and/or hypertensive. Cigarette smoking is an important risk factor which is increasing in young women as a result of 'clever' targeted advertising against a background of increasing social pressure. Hyperlipidaemia should be looked for; but the full lipid profile must always be measured as women have a higher HDL until the age of 65 years, and lowering this will be counterproductive. The low-dose contraceptive pills do not appear to increase the incidence of CAD, though smoking while on the pill is a cause for concern and should always be counselled against.

Women benefit from treatment the same as men but are often older at presentation and with more severe disease; this combined with naturally smaller coronary arteries may contribute to the slightly higher complication and mortality rate noted for PTCA and CABG.

Hormone replacement therapy (HRT) appears to lower the incidence of CAD by 50 per cent. Studies, however, are observational and no prospective trials have been completed. The possibility arises that women at low risk — higher social classes and 'healthy' women in general — self-select themselves for HRT which distorts the perceived benefit from HRT. However, it is difficult to ignore a 50 per cent reduction; it must be remembered that this relates to oral oestrogen only and, though CAD is reduced, overall mortality is not affected. We have no information on progestagens.

HRT should be considered for those post-menopausal women with established CAD and for those with a strong family history or major risk factors for CAD. Women need a full explanation of the pros and cons. The risk of breast cancer is small; nonetheless, women with a strong family history of breast cancer should probably not take HRT.

Women do not always receive the same treatment as men for a given cardiac problem. The question of a sex bias is disputed but is almost certainly real, though there is always the possibility of age bias (women are older at presentation).

Specific areas

Unstable angina
Variant angina
Chest pain with normal coronary arteries
Practical points

Unstable angina

Unstable angina has been defined on page 7. To summarize: it is angina at rest or minimal exertion without ECG or enzyme evidence of infarction. Unstable angina is a volatile and dangerous condition reflecting fissuring of an atheromatous plaque, thrombosis and possibly spasm. Mortality is high (20 per cent at 1 month) in those who fail to respond to medical treatment and is greater in those with previous angina, infarction or abnormal ECGs.

As the distribution and severity of the coronary lesions as well as the presence of LV dysfunction determine prognosis, in suitable patients angiography within two weeks is advised (Figure 15).

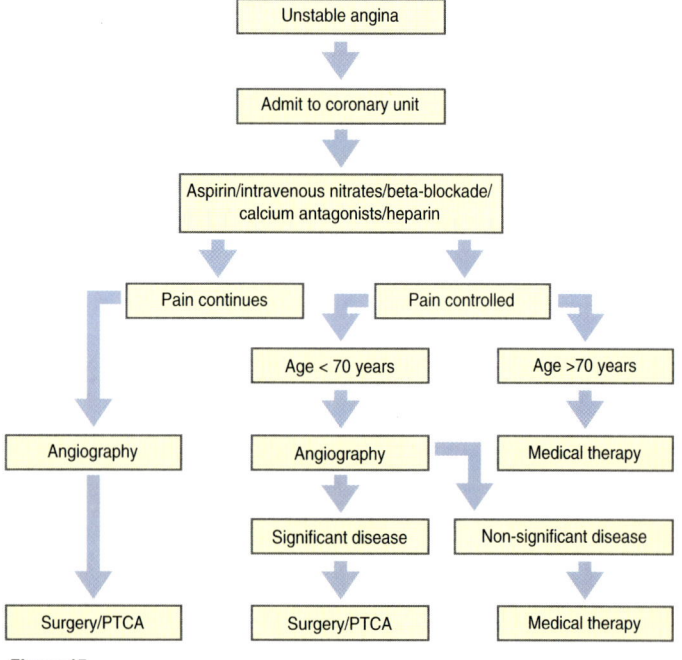

Figure 15
Unstable angina management plan.

Management is aimed at:

- Relief of symptoms

- Prevention of infarction

- Survival.

Immediate care

Out of hospital:

- Sublingual nitrates and iv opiates, plus 300 mg of aspirin for platelet effects (chewed for rapid onset of action).

In hospital (coronary care unit supervision and monitoring is necessary):

- Begin iv nitrates using isosorbide dinitrate 2 mg/hour, titrating to pain relief and keeping systolic blood pressure >100 mmHg.
- Begin heparin infusion (30 000–40 000 units/day): monitor to keep partial thromboplastin time 2–3 x control (continue for 24–48 hours).
- Continue aspirin 300 mg 12-hourly for 2 days.
- Begin beta-blockade if not contraindicated: eg, atenolol 50 mg orally or 5 mg slowly iv if pain with tachycardia continues. The alternative is diltiazem 60–120 mg tds. Add nifedipine retard to beta-blockade if pain continues but do not use as monotherapy (amlodipine is not currently indicated for unstable angina).
- If there is any suggestion of infarction give thrombolytic drugs.
- If pain continues in spite of the above, refer for immediate angiography with a view to PTCA or CABG.

	Prevents Angina	Prevents Infarction
β-blockers	Yes	Possibly
Calcium channel blockers	Yes	Unproven
Intravenous nitroglycerin and nitrates	Yes	Unproven
Heparin	Probably	Yes
Aspirin	No	Yes
Thrombolytic therapy	No	No
Coronary angioplasty	Yes	No
Coronary bypass surgery	Yes	No

Table 12
Effect of therapy for unstable angina

When the patient is stable

- Switch to oral mononitrate 20–40 mg bid and wean off iv nitrates
- Continue beta-blockade and/or calcium antagonist
- Continue aspirin now at 75 mg day
- Wean off heparin
- If age < 70 years arrange angiography before discharge. Over 70 manage on mobility and symptoms. (Do not be too arbitrary about age — consider biological age as well as actual age)
- Use elective PTCA/CABG for appropriate lesions as prognostic benefits have been established.

Variant angina

'Variant angina' refers to patients who get pain at rest with ST elevation on the ECG. It may occur at the same time of day (the most common being night and early morning) and be associated with syncope. Exertional angina may or may not coexist.

The cause is coronary artery spasm. There was a 9 per cent death rate and a 38 per cent infarct rate at two years in Prinzmetal's series. If the coronary anatomy is normal, cardiac events occur in 8 per cent; if CAD exists, cardiac events occur in 30 per cent.

These (old) figures may be influenced by newer drugs and techniques.

Management

A management strategy is shown in Figure l6.

Note that nitrates and calcium antagonists are first-choice agents. The condition should be managed initially as unstable angina. Existing beta-blockade should be continued, especially if CAD is known; it should be avoided otherwise (the unopposed alpha effects may lead to vasoconstriction). Aspirin should be used as for unstable angina.

When the angina is stable proceed to angiography. If significant CAD exists atenolol may be added at this point. CABG has a higher risk here than for stable angina, and spasm may recur post-operatively. Continue anti-spasm drugs post-operatively (eg, diltiazem plus mononitrates). If there is refractory spasm insert an aortic balloon pump in addition to drug therapy (this is very rarely needed).

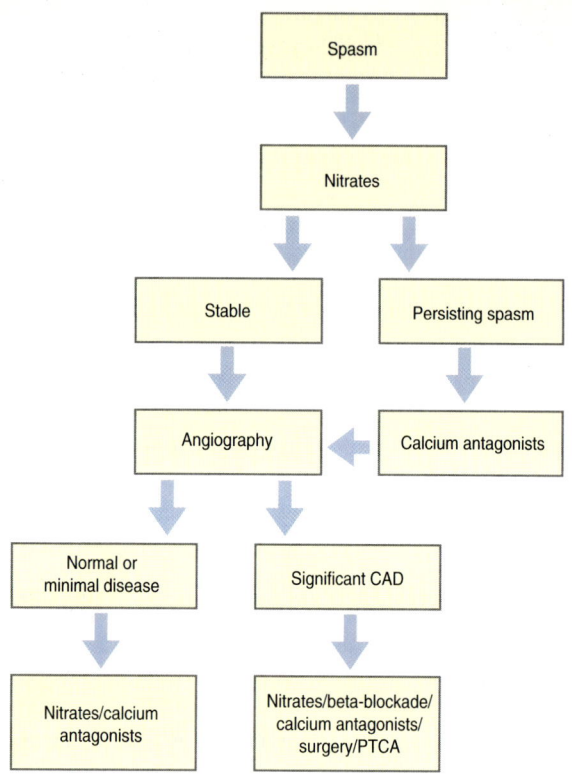

Figure 16
Variant angina management plan.

Chest pain with normal coronary arteries

This is a difficult group to manage. The incidence is higher in women — about 40 per cent compared to 5 per cent in men. The prognosis is excellent but the morbidity worrying.

Syndrome X relates to chest pain with NCA and typical pain with ST depression on exercise.

- Mortality at 10 years < 1 per cent
- Infarction incidence < 1 per cent
- Continuing pain 75 per cent
- 50 per cent unemployed or disabled.

In those with non-cardiac pain or atypical pain or no clear evidence of ischaemia it is important to rule out:

- Hyperventilation
- Oesophageal reflux or motility disorder
- Psychological illness (58–70 per cent of cases).

Treatment can be very problematic. Reassurance concerning prognosis is essential. Try to withdraw cardiac drugs to reinforce the normality in the angiogram but if they are continued for hypertension, say why this is, to avoid appearing contradictory.

Typical pain and abnormal ST changes may respond to conventional anti-anginal therapy. Anti-depressants may help selected cases. Women may benefit from oestrogen.

Practical points

Stable angina

- Treating angina is a team approach between patient and doctor.
- Symptoms can be controlled with nitrates, beta-blockers and calcium antagonists.
- Most nitrates are subject to hepatic metabolism but this can be avoided by using a mononitrate preparation.
- Beta-blockade needs to be used to optimal dose and not reduced when asymptomatic resting bradycardia occurs.
- When beta-blockers are contraindicated, use calcium antagonists and/or nitrates.
- Peripheral side-effects of beta-blockers can be reduced by dose reduction, using an agent with PAA or changing to calcium antagonists.
- Amlodipine, diltiazem and verapamil are effective as monotherapy. Nifedipine and amlodipine by avoiding conduction interaction are safer and effective in combination with beta-blockade, whereas diltiazem can be used cautiously in combination (verapamil is not recommended).
- Most adverse effects are caused by inappropriate patient selection; do not take chances.
- Angioplasty is successful in 90 per cent of patients but 30 per cent relapse at 6 months. If successful at 6 months, the long-term benefit is encouraging.
- PTCA is more effective than medical therapy for single lesions and moderate angina.

- Stents may reduce restenosis post PTCA and are more effective for vein graft lesions.
- Surgery is more effective than PTCA in relieving symptoms with less reintervention long term.
- Surgery not only prolongs life for some but relieves symptoms in 80 per cent of those failing to respond to medicine.
- Age should be no barrier to surgery if the patient is otherwise well.
- Surgical mortality averages 2 per cent. For the family, however, a death is 100 per cent.
- Aspirin (75 mg) is advised for all suitable cases.

Unstable angina

- Unstable angina is effort pain of recent onset, a changing pattern of angina or angina at rest.
- Hospital admission is advised.
- Intravenous nitrates form the mainstay of therapy.
- Beta-blockade and calcium antagonists can be added and should be continued if the patient is admitted already taking them.
- Aspirin, if not contraindicated, is begun immediately.
- Heparin should be infused for 24–48 hours.
- Angiography is advised, to rule out significant disease needing angioplasty or surgery.

Variant angina

- Coronary artery spasm may occur with and without CAD.
- It is the cause of variant angina.
- It is involved in 30–40 per cent of cases of unstable angina.
- The most rapidly effective drugs are the intravenous nitrates.
- Calcium antagonists are frequently helpful, alone or in combination with nitrates.
- Angiography is advised to rule out significant coronary disease.
- If surgery is performed spasm may still recur, so nitrates and calcium antagonists may be used post-operatively, even if the patient is apparently pain-free.

Often overlooked

- CAD occurs in premenopausal women also.
- Lipids need monitoring.
- The effect on the family — need for rehabilitation and support.
- The effect on the children of parents with heart disease.

Index

A

accelerated angina *see* unstable angina
acebutolol, 45, 46
acute coronary insufficiency *see* unstable angina
aetiology, stable angina, 16
age and incidence of coronary artery disease, 5
alcohol, 34, 36, 38
amlodipine, 47, 49, 50, 51–3, 71
anaemia, 16
anatomy, coronary, 29
angina
    causes, 11–12
    clinical evaluation, 16–17, 30
    coronary angioplasty, 54–60
    coronary surgery, 61–3
    definitions, 6–7
    drug therapy, 39–53
    general management, 34–8
    grading, 7
    incidence, 4, 5
    investigations, 18–32
    prevention, 64–5
angina decubitus, 14
angiography, 22–3, 29–30
    unstable angina, 71, 72
angioplasty *see* percutaneous transluminal coronary angioplasty
anti-depressants, 75
aortic aneurysm, dissecting, 15
aortic balloon pump, 73
aortic valve disease, 16, 17
apical dyskinesia, 17
arrhythmias, 16, 26, 48, 49, 50
aspirin, 53, 58, 65, 71, 72, 73
atenolol, 43, 44–5, 46, 51–3, 71, 73
atherectomy, 59, 60
atrial fibrillation, 16

B

Benestent trial, 58–9
beta-blockers, 19, 21, 42–6
    adverse effects, 43–4
    cardioselective, 42
    combination therapy, 51–2, 53
    exercise testing, 24
    partial agonist activity, 42–3

    unstable angina, 71, 72
    use, 43
    variant angina, 73, 74
    withdrawal, 46
bisoprolol, 45
blood pressure, 32
bradycardia, 52–3
breathlessness, 11, 15
bronchospasm, 48
bruits, 17

C

calcium antagonists, 46–51
    adverse effects, 48–9
    combination therapy, 51–3
    exercise testing, 24
    properties, 47
    unstable angina, 71, 72
    use, 47–50
    variant angina, 73, 74
chest pain
    causes, 11–12
    character, 6, 11
    diagnosis, 8–15
    myocardial infarction, 15
    nocturnal, 26, 41
    non-cardiac causes, 14–15
    with normal coronary arteries, 75
    radiation, 8
    relief, 13
    site, 8–10
    women, 12–13, 75
chest wall pain, 8, 9
cholesterol, 31, 35–8, 64
    effect of beta-blockers, 44
cholestyramine, 38
cigarette smoking *see* smoking
ciprofibrate, 38
clinical evaluation, stable angina, 16–17
colestipol, 38
contraceptive pill, 66
coronary anatomy, 29
coronary angiography, 22–3, 29–30, 71, 72
coronary angioplasty *see* percutaneous transluminal coronary angioplasty
coronary artery bypass grafting (CABG), 18, 61–3
    comparison with PTCA, 56–7, 61, 62
    indications, 63